Finding
The
Bright
Side

Actively seeking and finding
the bright side of
Alzheimer's Disease

Always look for the bright side!
Marlene Krafft Beckner

Marlene Krafft Beckner

Finding the Bright Side

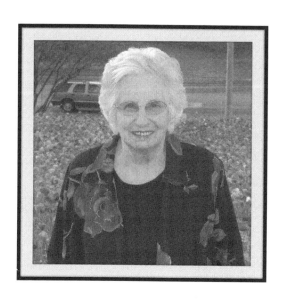

**In memory of my mother,
Alice Marjorie Brewer Weeks
January 23, 1925
to
December 19, 2009**

FOREWORD
by
Robert L. Alderman,
Minister at Large
Shenandoah Baptist Church, Roanoke,
Virginia

Alzheimer's is a frightening disease. When Marlene Beckner faced it in the life of her Mother she decided to face it with courage and victory instead of denial, defeat or desertion. She then decided to share the story with us.

Finding the Bright Side is the story of the journey Marlene took with her Mother, Alice. The details are not all pleasant. Some of those details are presented here with the stress and distress that accompany this disease. But there is more here.

In *Finding the Bright Side* Marlene reveals an attitude and insights that are refreshing and informative. That attitude models an informative example for all who must deal as care-givers and counselors with reference to the Alzheimer's situation. All of us who fall into the categories of the concerned, the care-giver or the counselor should read this story.

Here also is a word of encouraging insight. Marlene and her Mother, Alice, entered this journey with an informed relationship with Christ. They knew the assurance of abundant and eternal life with Christ. They knew that not even Alzheimer's could separate them from "the love of Christ." They knew the promise that in Christ they were "more than conquerors." (Romans 8:35, 37)

With promises like that they entered the journey through Alzheimer's in the Light, and that is where they finished it - on *The Bright Side.*

Preface

I am the quintessential optimist. If asked the age-old question, "Is the glass half full or half empty" I would most likely reply with, "Actually, I think it's a little *more* than half full!" I say that just to give you a glimpse into who I am as a person and how I typically view life. Another thing that defines me as a person is my zeal for learning all I can about any new thing that comes into my life. This can sometimes be a handicap as I tend to saturate myself with a topic and don't always maintain a proper balance with the constants in my life. Now that you know two facts about me, let me delve into my subject matter.

In my ongoing education about Alzheimer's disease and how it affects all whose life it touches, I discovered a gap in reading material. I found many helpful resources that cover all aspects of Alzheimer's disease from the diagnosis to the final stages and everything in between. There are even resources available to aid in adapting your home to accommodate a person with the diagnosis of Alzheimer's disease. Two of the things I gleaned from my studies were: things will never "get better" and each stage is worse than the one before. These statements are self-fulfilling. The longer a person lives with Alzheimer's disease, the further away they go. I made a conscious decision: If each stage gets worse, then I must be grateful for today and celebrate what is good about today. Each day there must surely be something to be thankful for. I cannot resolve myself to think, "All that is Alzheimer's is dark."

There must be a bright side somewhere. After drawing that conclusion, that is where I found the gap – I haven't found anything that addresses the bright side of Alzheimer's disease. I gaze out my window to a dark world and just as

Finding the Bright Side

I am sure that the sun is shining somewhere right now, I am sure there is a bright side to the dark disease called "Alzheimer's." I am now on a quest to find that bright side.

Let me now introduce you to the person I know whose life this disease has altered – my mother, Alice Marjorie Brewer Weeks. She has always been a strong woman with grit and determination. If it was in her heart to do something, her head would figure out a way to do it. She raised three girls – sometimes single-handedly. It never occurred to me that one day she wouldn't recognize these girls she had raised. And without knowing it, she built into the three of us what we would need in order to provide the same loving care to her that she had provided to us. She taught us that we had an amazing inner strength. She taught us about the God that we would need to call upon when we had no more strength of our own. She taught us how to live a life of grace even in the worst of circumstances. She taught us how to make do when there was nothing to do with.

She unknowingly taught us how to care for our mother as we observed the way she cared for her own mother. I will be forever grateful for the things I learned at my mother's side. And now I will share with you the things I am currently learning as I choose to stay by my mother's side. I will endeavor to show you the bright side of life. You can find the dark side somewhere else.

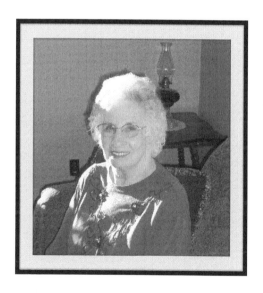

Acknowledgements

As I have accompanied my mother on this journey called, "Alzheimer's Disease" I must say we were joined by many wonderful people on this path. In reading this book, please do not get the idea that it was just my mother and me. I would like to thank the special people in our lives who have joined us on this journey.

To my husband, Daryl – Your kind heart and generous spirit have sustained me thru the most difficult time of our lives. You are without a doubt the most patient man I have ever known. Thank you for your tender care of my beloved mother.

To my son, Darren and his family – I have grieved over the time I have lost in your lives. You will never know how much I have enjoyed the times spent with you here in our home when I couldn't go out. Thank you Lauren, for planning activities when I couldn't begin to plan.

To my daughter, Emily – You have been such fun for Nana! She loved your teasing! You have stepped up and made life more convenient for us all. You have shouldered a lot of responsibility. Thank you for helping get your sister to various activities and for all the trips to Walmart when I couldn't get out to go shopping!

To my daughter, Lizzy – I realize all of your teen years and even prior to that, you have had to share your mother way too much. In spite of that, you have turned into an amazing person. Thank you for always being an encouragement to me.

To my sister, Michelle – You have helped me find the bright side many times in life. Your indomitable spirit has been an inspiration to me. Thank you for the many times you have come in and told me, "I'm here, you're off the clock now!"

To my sister, Yvonne – You have made so many sacrifices and traveled so many miles to help take care of Mom. I am sure none of us know the true toll this has taken on you. Thank you for your willing spirit to help in any way you could.

To my nephew, John Clint – You have been such a great joy to Nana. You have always been kind to her and considerate of her. She loved looking at the beautiful rocks you decorated. Thank you for always being so willing to help out when called upon.

To my nephew, Shaun – You know how special you have always been to Nana. You were the apple of her eye. You have done a fantastic job of carrying on her beach legacy! Thank you and Mindi for all of the fun visits and for bringing laughter with you every time!

To my Uncle Max and Aunt Becky – You have traveled from Walnut Cove, NC so many times to visit Mom and she always enjoyed your visits so much. It was always a joy to see you. Thank you for being such a wonderful brother and sister-in-law to Mom.

To my father-in-law and mother-in-law, Buster and Pat – Mom always enjoyed your lively visits! You always had something fun to talk about! Thank you for the many times you came and sat with Mom so Daryl and I could go out.

To my grandmother-in-law, Nelda – God's providence brought you to our home the last couple of months of Mom's life. She enjoyed your companionship and I appreciate the way you "looked after her."

To our dear friend, Phyllis – You have been so faithful to call and check on Mom and to visit so regularly. We all enjoyed your visits and want you to know we'll still put on a pot of coffee any time you want to stop by! Thank you for the way you have loved our whole family thru the years.

To our dear friend, Shirley – You originally touched our lives through music, and we have all learned so much through you. You have been a great blessing to us as we see you live your life in harmony with God's Word. Thank you for always remembering Mom with the beautiful roses.

To our special friend, Virginia – You invited Mom to church in 1967 where she heard the Gospel message and trusted in Christ as her personal savior. God used you to change the course of her life and that of many generations.

To our dear friends, Jim, Deb and Norma – You have been such an example to me in the way you cared for Kiah. You traveled this path before me and helped me find my way. Thank you for being such an encouragement to me over the years.

To Mom's wonderful physician, Dr. Richard Newton, Sr. – Besides being a top notch cardiologist, you are a true southern gentleman and we all greatly admire and respect you. Thank you for the good, attentive care you have given to Mom over the years.

To our Pastors and fellow members of Shenandoah Baptist Church – you have been so faithful to pray for Mom through the years. We have been so blessed to be part of this church family. Thank you for the visits and notes letting us know of your prayers on our behalf.

To Good Samaritan Hospice – You have been such a blessing in our lives by helping us in the practical areas of life. Thank you Jean, Amber, Bridget, Alice, and Shirley for partnering with us to make it easier to care for Mom here at home.

To the Alzheimer's Association local chapter – Annette, Margaret and Maggie, you ladies are awesome! I feel like we bonded immediately and my heart is knit with yours as we care for our loved ones. Thank you for being such an encouragement and inspiration to me!

To my readers

As you read through this book, please keep in mind that events were written in chronological order. You will see a natural progression of Alzheimer's Disease. Skills that are present one day are not necessarily present the next.

And always remember, "When you've seen one person with Alzheimer's Disease, you've seen **one person** with Alzheimer's Disease." Your journey will be different, but my prayer is that no matter where the journey takes you, you will find the bright side.

Author's Disclaimer

Author has no prior experience with Alzheimer's disease; nor does she have a medical background. These writings are strictly based on first-hand (learn as you go) experience.

I noticed a number of months ago that when I asked my Mom if she needed anything from the store – she would look in the bathroom to see if she had "Poise pads" and denture cleaning supplies. Had her life been reduced to this? Were those her only perceived needs?

The bright side: She has a confident feeling of being well cared for and all of her needs are being met. She knows she will be provided with plenty to eat and someone else will remember to purchase her favorite snacks. The lesson I've learned from her short list of needs is: Do I really "need" all those things in life I strive for? As I ponder that question my list of "needs" keeps getting shorter and shorter.

In the past, Mom loved to buy new clothes. She loved vibrant colors. But now, she tends to wear the same outfit day after day. While she is in the kitchen eating breakfast I sometimes go into her room and retrieve the outfit she has worn two or three days in a row so I can wash it.

The bright side: She still tends to gravitate towards the brighter items in her closet thereby showing me that she is still the same person that she always was with her same likes and dislikes. It is now my privileged responsibility to remember her preferences and honor her by honoring them. Another thing to be thankful for: She can see to choose her favorite colors, she can still make that choice even if she can't make other choices and she can still dress herself. There's always something to be thankful for!

Mom has withdrawn from her previous activities and has to be encouraged to engage in meaningful activities.

The bright side: Because of Mom's diagnosis, I have greatly reduced the amount of activities I participate in outside the home. Perhaps I'm learning that I don't need all the busy-ness that I once proclaimed was so important. There are a few activities I'd really like to engage in but this is just not my season of life to enjoy those things. When the time comes to re-join society so to speak, I'll have an increased awareness of what is important to me as an individual and to my family as a whole and will be better fitted to make wise decisions about how I invest my time. Thank you Mom for teaching me another valuable life lesson.

There are so many activities around the home that Mom no longer remembers how to do.

The bright side: She still remembers how to vacuum and whenever she doesn't know what to do with herself and wants to contribute somehow, she'll say, "Can I vacuum the kitchen?" Our floors have never looked better! Thanks Mom!

Mom doesn't always recognize this place called home.

The bright side: Even though she doesn't realize this is the same home she has lived in for 43 years, she knows she loves it here and says so on a daily basis. She often asks if she can stay here forever. Of course I say yes, and then remind her that this is home. She is always so happy when she "discovers" this is actually her home.

Mom forgets new information whether it's good news or bad news.

The bright side: Every time we tell her the same good news, she's always just as happy to hear it as she was the first time she heard it! On the flip side: we don't repeat bad news so she only has to grieve once.

In addition to forgetting current happenings, I've noticed Mom has forgotten many past experiences.

The bright side: I always listened carefully to the family stories Mom told of her years growing up and of her young adulthood - stories of her brothers, her parents, her grandparents, her work experiences. Now she listens just as attentively to me as I retell to her the same stories she has told me through the years. These stories bring much joy to her and sometimes a spark of recognition will ignite into a glowing flame as some of the memories come back to her and she will join in the retelling of the stories.

I could never understand how Alzheimer's disease could rob a formerly active person of so many thoughts.

The bright side: Mom used to be so busy – many times she was too busy to enjoy the simple things of life – the gifts God gives us each day that we awaken. Now Mom "lives in the moment". Her mind is not cluttered up with responsibilities, millions of past memories, concerns for the future. I could not begin to tell you the number of times in the past few months that she has said, "We live in a beautiful world." I think she sees and appreciates like never before the wonders that God has created for us to enjoy.

I have read that Alzheimer's disease sometimes alters sleep patterns. This seems to be the case for Mom. Whereas she used to retire early, now she stays up so late.

The bright side: She is an adult in her own home and can go to bed whenever she pleases! She has earned that right. No one is going to tell her "lights out!" Granted, we may ask her doctor to prescribe a sleep aid for her so that WE can get some sleep!

In the past, Mom was always a germ freak. She was so afraid we'd "get a germ!" Clorox was her best friend. Now she wants to wash the dishes, dry them and put them in the cabinet without the dishes ever seeing a drop of soap...unclean!! No amount of prodding will convince her that those dishes cannot possibly be clean without the use of dish liquid.

The bright side: She taught me to be a germ freak as well so now to protect our health, I try to keep the dishes washed and put away or at least loaded into the dishwasher where they are safe! And, it's given me a new appreciation for the good job our immune system does when it keeps us from "getting a germ!"

Mom has been known to hold a grudge. We all have our faults so I don't feel disloyal for naming this as one of her's. Usually it would take a great deal of injustice to raise her ire to the point that she wouldn't let go of it but there have been a few things in her life that she's been bitter about and carried that around for many years.

The bright side: Holding a grudge would involve remembering the person who wronged you or at least the incident that caused hurt. As she seems to travel further and further down that road of memory loss, those few grudges that she carried around with her seem to be laid by the wayside, forgotten, never to be picked up again. She is now completely free of those burdens that once weighed her down.

She often doesn't remember us – her three daughters who love and care for her, her grandchildren whom she's known and loved, her friends who have always respected her so highly.
The bright side: She doesn't have to remember us – we remember her – and that is enough.

I will admit, this morning it was hard to think of the bright side of this one for a few minutes. I am so tired because for some unknown reason, Mom stayed awake last night – all night long. She fiddled with her things in her room (packing I assume) all night long. At 5am, she yelled out my name and I jumped out of bed in a fright to see what was wrong. She wanted to know where everyone was. I said, "Everyone's in bed – it's the middle of the night." I asked her if she'd been to bed yet and she said "No!" I encouraged her to go back to bed but could tell via the audio monitor that she continued to arrange her things until after Daryl, my husband left for work at 8:30. (She's now sleeping, but of course I'm not.)

The bright side: My schedule isn't so hectic these days so I may be able to catch a nap later.

Mom frequently brings me a framed photograph of her mother that dates back to the 1920's.

It is a beautiful portrait and has always been admired by anyone who sees it. Mom often asks if she "can have that picture to give to her mother." The first time Mom asked me that, I assured her that the picture already belongs to her and that Grandma is in heaven now. Oh, the heartbreaking experience of seeing my mother weep as if being told this news for the first time. And in fact I believe it was worse than the first time she heard it, because when she dwelt in the land of reality, she knew Grandma's passing was imminent and although she grieved, she accepted her death. This time however, it was a real shock to her as she "learned" of her mother's death. The corresponding questions I was called to answer between her tears and mine were so difficult. This was *her mother* whom she loved and cherished and she came to the full realization that her mother was gone from her. That was one of the hardest moments to date that I have endured in this journey. I comforted her in her grief, answered her questions, assured her of the promises in God's Word that she would one day see her mother again and then began reminding her of precious memories of her mother.

The bright side: I learned a valuable lesson that night: A mother's love is never forgotten. She may have forgotten the fact that her mother had graduated to heaven; she may have forgotten the fact that she had already grieved for her; but she did not forget the fact that she and her mother shared a special kind of love. When she realized she had lost her mother, she knew it was a terrible thing. The distinct memories of her mother may have faded from my Mom's brain, but the lasting impression of a mother's love is indelibly imprinted on her heart.

The past few days, Mom's struggles as well as other burdens that I carry began to overwhelm me. Yesterday I felt like a piece of shattered glass just before it falls from its casing. A tap of a fingernail against the glass would be enough to send it pouring in a heap to the floor. Today I compare myself to a plain terra cotta pot that has broken into chunks and has been pieced back together with duct tape - unsightly but functional. Not a very pretty picture. My nerves were frayed and my tears would not stop.

The bright side: The tears eventually did stop and during the tears I learned several lessons. First lesson: I am fragile right now and I need to be kind to myself. Second lesson: I need to get my eyes off myself and back on the Lord "from whence cometh my help." Third lesson: The Lord let me have a glimpse into my heart and it was a much uglier picture than my mind had conceived. However, God in His goodness did not leave me in my despair. He drew me to repentance so I could have a clean heart before Him and a renewed desire to please Him in all I am and in all I do. Fourth lesson: I was reminded that I need to give my burdens to the Lord daily, hourly if needed!

Today Mom came to me with a confused, concerned look on her face that I couldn't quite discern. I asked her if she was ok, and she said no. She whispered to me what she needed to do and that she didn't know where to do it. I pointed her to the bathroom and she was greatly relieved to see that was exactly where she needed to be!

The bright side: At least she asked! Enough said on that subject.

Mom requires total assistance to take a shower now. By the time "we" are finished, the floor is soaked and I am almost as wet as she is!

The bright side: The bathroom floor can always stand a good mopping!

The other day Mom didn't remember where to use the bathroom but the bright side was – at least she asked. Well, today she didn't ask! Oops!

The bright side: Took me a minute to think of the bright side of this one as I was cleaning out her bedside potty. After disinfecting it, I realized I was thankful that at least she used her potty rather than less desirable options. It really could have been worse. And at least I found "it" right away! ☺ I read a quote by Marie Osmond yesterday that prepared me for today's challenge, "If you're going to be able to look back on something and laugh about it, you might as well laugh about it now."

More often than not, Mom does not have a clue as to who I am.

The bright side: She loves/likes me anyway! Every night when I tuck her in, she thanks me for my "goodness to her and my kindness to her." This morning she said, "You know, I really like you!" I can't think of a finer compliment!

Even though we've been on this journey well over 2 years, as a caregiver it scares me when I realize we haven't gotten to the really difficult challenges of Alzheimer's Disease.

The bright side: The Holy Bible supplies many admonitions to refrain from worrying about the future and many assurances that he will supply the grace needed when it's needed. I am so thankful for God's Word that is living and powerful! It becomes dearer to me with each passing day.

Mom has begun having hallucinations. It doesn't happen all the time, but when it does, the images are so very real to her. She hears strange noises and sees spiders, toads, unfamiliar people and sometimes pouring rain.

The bright side: I am so grateful that we are able to be right here with her so her fears can be quickly addressed. But how do I respond to her when she sees things that I don't see and hears things that I don't hear? Maybe the same way she responded to me when I was a child and I saw and heard things that she didn't see or hear. She gently reassured me, brushed away my fears and asked me if I was alright now.

Mom woke this morning totally confused about her surroundings. Nothing looked familiar to her and no amount of prodding brought back any memories of her home. I even referred to the beloved dogs in the back yard and the cats on the porch and she didn't remember any of it. I finally showed her pictures of our house, pointing out the mail box by the front door, her rocking chair on the front porch, and still nothing was familiar to her. She had no recollection of this place and long after breakfast, she still kept saying she's never been so confused in her life. "I'm just lost" she said as she looked at me with beseeching eyes that begged me to help her find her way again.

The bright side: Remembering a helpful idea I learned from a dear friend who's walked this path before me, I purposefully took Mom out for ice-cream just so we could drive home. As we approached our house, I asked, "Who lives here?" She exclaimed, "WE DO!" ...My Mama found her way once again.

Mom still does not recognize this house as being her home. In the past, I've been able to tell her that this is her home and she would be so happy to hear that good news. But now, months have passed and reminding her that this is home is no longer any comfort to her. In her heart and mind, home has transitioned to a place from days gone by. Whether it's an exact location or particular loved ones she is longing for I cannot tell, but her perceived reality tells her *this place is not home.*

That perception leads her to become extremely homesick. If we are unsuccessful at our attempts to distract her from this feeling, she becomes agitated.

The bright side: God is not surprised at this development. It is not a new concept with Him. In fact, scriptures tell us to long for our heavenly home. Maybe Mom is not too far off track in longing for a home where her loved ones abide.

Mom has required round the clock care and/or monitoring since June, 2006. This means Daryl and I usually do not attend church together as one or the other stays home with her.

The bright side: On occasion, one of my sisters is able to be with Mom on Sunday so Daryl and I can worship together. We treasure those times and no longer take for granted the privilege of worshipping God together.

The other day Mom was participating in a peculiar activity. She had bunched up a tissue and then bunched up the ribbon from her housecoat with it, and was attempting to cut the ribbon off her housecoat with fingernail clippers. I was so distressed to observe this unexplainable behavior. It seemed she was out of her mind doing something so bizarre.

The bright side: God quickened my spirit to realize this activity harkened back to her days as a florist when she probably tied a million bows! She was gathering the white tissue and white ribbon up together as if tying a lovely bow and of course she needed to cut the ribbon!   Now it made perfect sense!   We turned that "strange" action into a craft project and I assisted her to make beautiful tissue paper flowers in bright colors! She now has a hobby that she loves and she can share her flowers with others!!

Last summer I had a small vegetable garden that included a few tomato plants. I watched carefully as the plants grew and the tomatoes began to form on the vine. I looked forward to that day when I could pick our first vine ripe tomato of the season. Evidently Mom had been watching those plants too; however, orange tomatoes striped with green were evidently appealing to her as she picked "my" first tomato about 3 days before it was ripe. All summer she proceeded to pick the tomatoes a few days before they were ripe and proudly placed them in the kitchen window to ripen! They were a trophy to her, but a source of contention to me. I was ashamed of myself for being aggravated, but aggravated I was, plain and simple! I am still ashamed of my attitude about those tomatoes last summer. I realized we had a conflict with her actions and my attitude. How would we handle that situation this summer?

The bright side: I know God placed this idea in my heart....this year I planted little cherry tomatoes near the house so Mom can pick tomatoes to her heart's content. The larger variety are further away from the house where she won't notice them on a daily basis and I can walk with her out to that part of the garden when they are ripe and ready to be picked!

Mom was hospitalized this weekend, and whether it was from exhaustion or from being in a strange place, she became very combative. In the night, she became angry with me as well as her nurse, swinging punches and saying terrible things. We have never experienced this before, and after the episode was over and Mom was asleep, I sobbed with grief.

The bright side: This one is for you, my brothers and sisters who have walked this road before me with your loved one. I prayed for you that night. I may not know you, but I prayed for those who have had to witness this heart-breaking transformation and those of you who have yet to experience it. It was the hardest night of my life but God brought me through and he will bring me thru again. I am not alone.

While in the hospital, Mom was diagnosed with Stage 5 kidney failure. Dr. Newton, her primary physician and cardiologist, knows Mom well and knows our desire to care for her no matter what. His recommendation was that we bring Mom home with hospice and offer comfort measures and help her live out her days surrounded by those who love her. We are following his recommendation but when that ambulance backed up to the ramp leading to our porch, and I saw my mother sitting in the back of that ambulance, all I could think of was, "This is the day they are bringing my Mama home to die." I had to turn away so she wouldn't see my tears. I will never forget that image of her sweet, smiling face as she began the end of her journey. Writing these words causes a new wave of grief to wash over me.

The bright side: How many times in life do we have the opportunity to show those we care about how much we love them? All the time, opportunities abound. How many times do we take advantage of those opportunities? Not nearly enough. I am more keenly aware than ever the importance of showing and telling my loved ones what they mean to me. Not just my mom, but my sisters, my husband, my children, my granddaughter and everyone else I care about.

Mom is experiencing an overall decline. One indication of this decline is the fact that she is becoming incontinent. I had dreaded the disease taking us to this stage. For her I dreaded the use of "adult diapers" and the stigma attached to their use. For myself, I had dreaded the inconvenience and added responsibility that this stage of Alzheimer's disease would require from me.

The bright side: There are so many products available these days to help with this problem. We found a wonderful product that pulls on just like the undergarments she was used to wearing and she doesn't even question when I assist her. It was a very smooth transition for her and it actually lightens my load as I'm not required to change sheets every morning!

Mom's perception of time is skewed. If I am out of her sight for more than a moment, she looks for me, thinking I've been gone for a long time. It puts quite a bit of pressure on me. It matters not if I've just stepped into the bathroom or around the corner to the laundry room, she will come looking for me, and when she "finds" me, she'll say, "Oh, there you are! I thought I'd lost you!"

The bright side: Mom is still mobile and can navigate thru the house. I am thankful that she can still walk and is able to search for me.

It is impossible to get a good night's sleep to prepare us for the coming day. Even if Mom's door alarm doesn't wake me, indicating she has left her room, I find myself waking during the night to listen for her, unable to determine if she is still tucked safely in her bed.

The bright side: I discovered a video monitor advertised for use in monitoring babies. It turned out to be a wonderful purchase! Now when I wake, I can check the monitor beside my bed and actually see if she is still sleeping. If so, I can drift back off to sleep without having to go downstairs to check on her. I have slept much better since finding this wonderful device!

Mom has been very pleasant throughout her illness. However there have been some times that she has been "not so pleasant!" Such as when she says, "Shut up!" or "Leave me alone!" or "You are driving me crazy!" That doesn't happen often, but when it does, it's difficult to remember that it's the disease, not my mother talking.

The bright side: We have finally discovered the trigger that seems to precede every outburst. We discovered that if we mention anything about toileting in front of others, she becomes very upset. So now, rather than asking, "Would you like to go to the bathroom?" We say, "Let's take a walk." She very willingly receives assistance then.

Taking care of Mom requires a lot of bending and stooping as I help her get dressed and especially when I assist her in the bathroom. Often I will get down on my knees to help her lift her feet one at a time to put her undergarments back on. She has always been such a modest, private person and would be mortified if she knew how much personal care her daughters have had to administer on her behalf. One day she looked down at me and said, "You've had a lot of experience with this haven't you?"

The bright side: This is one time I was glad my mother didn't realize who I was. She was more comfortable receiving assistance from a "professional person", not realizing I was her own daughter. After she commented on my experience, I laughed and told her, "Yes, I've had lots of experience!" I think she was pleased that she had an "experienced" care-giver!

Many times these past few weeks, my mother has forgotten our exact relationship. She seems to have forgotten which one of us is the mother, and which one of us is the daughter. She has told people several times lately that I was HER mother.

The bright side: This speaks volumes to me. It makes me know she feels loved and cared for just as her mother always loved and cared for her. I don't care who she thinks I am as long as she is content.

Mom is now completely incontinent. I have been so fearful of this part of the journey. To be honest, I just didn't know how I would manage. I am not the nurse in the family; I have never dealt with this before. Now that we are here, I realize how much I had fretted over it.

The bright side: It's really o.k. I have eased into this role and it's really no big deal to just put on my gloves and deal with it!

Over the years, Mom has expressed a fear of dying. We knew she had assurance of heaven, but we didn't know how to respond when she told us she was afraid to die.

The bright side: Alzheimer's disease has completely removed that fear. She doesn't think about death, and never mentions those fears to us.

I knew when we began this journey that it would get harder and harder. We are now at the "hard part." Mom's health is declining, she requires more assistance with every aspect of life and it is very hard to care for her day in and day out.

The bright side: We can deal with hard. Mom taught us to be hard workers and to not quit just because something was hard. So, as long as it's just hard, we can do it. If it becomes impossible, then we will consider our options, but as long as it's just hard, **we can do hard**!

Mom has taken a turn for the worse. Her speech is garbled and she is showing other signs of a stroke. Her hospice nurse checked her and agreed that it seems she is having small strokes. Mom declines all offers of food or water. Her nurse suggested we call any who may want to visit with her before it is too late. Her brother and family drove up from North Carolina to visit and most of her grandchildren were able to visit with her.

The bright side: I am so thankful for the blessing of a loving family. We need each other and it such a comfort to know Mom is so loved.

Mom has shown some improvement, took a little nourishment, but still hasn't been able to leave her bed. She barely talks and sleeps most of the time. I called our church so one of the pastors could visit with her and offer words of comfort to her.

The bright side: When Pastor Crutchfield arrived, Mom perked up, joked with him and then joined with him as he sang "Joy to the World!" I know my jaw must have dropped at this sudden rally! I'm not sure who was more surprised and thrilled – her daughters or Pastor Crutchfield! I will say though, he definitely had a bounce in his step when he left her room!

It's been a little over a week since Mom began having strokes and took a definite turn for the worse. It has been a heartbreaking week as we've had to turn Mom to change her and she has cried out and begged us to just leave her alone. We knew we couldn't leave her unattended for her own good, but we certainly cried after we were finished and she was once again resting comfortably.

The bright side: Mom's memory is so impaired that once we were finished with our task, she immediately returned to a resting state. We take great comfort that she is not suffering any pain.

It is the Christmas season, but we certainly don't feel festive. Our beloved mother/grandmother is dying.

The bright side: There is true peace in sitting by her bedside. Christmas carols are playing quietly in the background; there is no "busy-ness"; there is just my mother quietly sleeping and the beautiful music of Christmas. There is time to reflect on her life and on what she means to me. I am so blessed to think not only of her earthly life, but also of eternal life as Christ's birth has a new and deeper meaning for me this Christmas season.

My beloved mother has ended her earthly journey.

The bright side: We have "walked her to Jesus" one step at a time knowing that "to be absent from the body is to be present with the Lord." And that my dear friend is the ultimate bright side.

Epilogue

It has been about 3 ½ years since my mother was diagnosed with Alzheimer's disease. I was privileged to watch my mother gain victory over that disease on December 19, 2009 at 2:08 a.m. I would like to share with you the amazing story of God's tender mercies as witnessed by myself and my 2 sisters...

On December 18, Mom took a distinct turn for the worse, and my sisters and I could tell Death was lurking around the corner, waiting to snatch our mother from us. Death did not know we were on a journey, walking her to Jesus one step at a time. We had the calm assurance that her life was in God's hands and when He was ready, He would receive her unto Himself.

"To be absent from the body is to be present with the Lord."

As Mom lived her last day on this earth, snow was quietly falling outside, beautiful harp music was playing in her room and I was so blessed to be by her side along with my two sisters. We ministered to our mother, speaking words of comfort to her, holding her hand and just desiring to be in her presence. As the evening advanced, snow continued to fall and the winter wonderland scene was framed by the picture window in her room. The multi-colored glow of her small Christmas tree completed the serene setting. Sometime during the night, Mom slipped into a coma and we knew we would be releasing her to Jesus very soon. We sat by her bed, memorizing her features, praying for her comfort and speaking loving words to her. We could sense Mom was struggling between the earthly desires of family and home and the heavenly desires of being called home to Jesus. Throughout the evening, we each told our dear mother through muffled sobs that it was alright to leave us. We would be ok. We would continue to love each other and look after each other, and she was free to join all those family members who had gone before. We spoke to her of her parents as well as her grandparents, aunts and uncles, brother, grandson, cousins and friends who were waiting to welcome her. As she continued to labor for each breath and her heart raced, we told her of Moses and David and Abraham and how she would share eternity with them. We told her that

Jesus Himself would welcome her into His kingdom. A little later, the ragged breaths suddenly stopped and we watched our Mother open her eyes wide and look up toward heaven. Her eyes were clear and bright – they had lost that cloudy look that we had become so familiar with and she no longer had that lost look that accompanied Alzheimer's disease. Her eyes literally sparkled, and then the most amazing thing happened – without moving her head, her eyes slowly moved to the left, paused a second, and then slowly moved back to center. She then gently closed her eyes, took two short breaths and was gone.

The Bible speaks of a great cloud of witnesses, and we feel God blessed us with the privilege of seeing our mother gaze upon her loved ones whom we imagine were standing shoulder to shoulder waiting to welcome her home. Our Mother, who nurtured us, loved us, and led us to Jesus, has now joined that great cloud of witnesses that will one day welcome us home.

While these past few years have been the most difficult of my life, I would not trade them for anything this world has to offer. In talking with a friend at the funeral home, I realized I had lived all but 10 years of my life with my mother. I am so thankful that I have been able to share so much of my life with her. I would like to think some of her qualities have rubbed off on me in those 39 years together!

My mother's earthly life is over but her story lives on in my heart. I have the blessed assurance that I will one day see my mother in heaven. If you do not have the peaceful assurance that you will one day be reunited with your loved ones, and would like to be assured of a place in heaven, you may pray this simple prayer, "God, I know that I am a sinner. I know that I deserve the consequences of my sin. However, I am trusting in Jesus Christ as my Savior. I believe that His death and resurrection provided for my forgiveness. I trust in Jesus and Jesus alone as my personal Lord and Savior. Thank you Lord, for saving me and for forgiving me! Amen!"

Appendix
In this section you will find some things that I found to be helpful on this journey. I share them with you for your benefit to use as you see fit.

A dear volunteer from hospice came every week for the last 6 months of Mom's life. She came prepared to talk, sing, read or just sit with Mom. She found her own common ground with my mother, but to help her catch a glimpse of the amazing person my mother is and to offer topics of conversation, I wrote the following for our volunteer:

Alice enjoys....

The beach! She's lived in Miami, Wilmington NC, Chesapeake and Norfolk and we take her to the beach at least once a year. In recent years, she's been to the following beaches in North Carolina: Carolina Beach, Kure Beach, Wrightsville Beach, Holden Beach, Oak

Island, and the Outer Banks. She's also enjoyed beaches in South Carolina: Myrtle Beach and Hilton Head.

Flowers! She is a retired florist. She and I started A & M Floral Gallery on Williamson Road. We sold the business in 1996, and it is still operating as Roanoke Floral Gallery. By the way, A & M stands for Alice and Marlene.

Her daughters! There are 3 of us...Michelle, the oldest, a nurse at Roanoke Memorial Hospital; Yvonne, the middle daughter, a pastor's wife in Pennsylvania; and Marlene, "the baby", lives here with Mom along with my husband and 2 teenage daughters, Emily and Lizzy. My son, Darren is married to Lauren and they have a girl (age 2) named Savannah.

Music! She plays the piano, organ and accordion. She likes to listen to various types of music and one of her favorite singers is Johnny Cash.

The Bible! She loves the word of God and taught a ladies' Sunday school class for many years at Calvary Baptist Church in Salem. She is now a member of Shenandoah Baptist Church.

Gardening! She helped can most of the jars displayed over our kitchen cabinets.

Birds! She loves to sit on the side porch and watch the birds at the bird feeder.

Our home! She has lived here for 43 years although she doesn't always remember this is home.

Reading! She enjoys looking at books, magazines and the newspaper.

~~~~~

We utilized several audio and video monitors throughout our home. We had an audio/video monitor in her room and 2 audio monitors in other rooms downstairs. During the night, I kept all the monitors on with the receivers in my room so I could sleep in my own bed and still maintain an awareness of her safety.

~~~~~

My husband installed door alarms on all of our exterior doors as well as Mom's bedroom door. This was particularly helpful at night.

~~~~~

We purchased a silver bracelet and had Mom's name, address and phone number engraved on it. Thankfully she never wandered out of our yard, but it gave us peace of mind in case she did. She loved looking at it and reading her name engraved on it.

~~~~~

On the computer, I compiled a list of Mom's current medications with dosage instructions. I took a list to her doctor visits and kept a list in the medicine cabinet. Whenever changes needed to be made, I was able to easily update the list and noted at the bottom of the page the date it was updated.

~~~~~

Daryl installed a lock on our medicine cabinet door so I never had to worry about Mom overdosing. We used two weekly pill containers that were labeled with her name as well as a.m. medications or p.m. medications. This was helpful to me so I could look at her containers and make sure I had administered her medications at any given time.

~~~~~

I highly recommend the Alzheimer's Association. I wish I had availed myself of this resource sooner. The support group meetings were a great source of encouragement to me. After I began attending the meetings, I realized Mom's journey may be unique to her, but there are still many similarities amongst people with the diagnosis of Alzheimer's disease and I could learn much from other caregivers.

~~~~~

Three books that I highly recommend:

The 36-hour Day, written by Nancy L. Mace, M.A. and Peter V. Rabins, M.D., M.P.H.

The Complete Guide to Alzheimer's Proofing Your Home, written by Mark L. Warner

Coach Broyles' Playbook for Alzheimer's Caregivers, written by Coach Frank Broyles

~~~~~

It is my hope and prayer that no matter where you are in life, you will always remember to look for the bright side. Some days it may be more difficult to see than others, but it's there. There is always something to be thankful for, some reason to hope, some person who needs you or some purpose to which you were born. God made only ONE of you and you are going to live this life only ONCE so you may as well live it on the bright side! If it is not in your nature to see the bright side of life, you may have to train yourself to look for it! When faced with your next challenge in life, take a moment to stop and ask yourself, "What's the bright side of this situation?" Do that a few hundred times and pretty soon it will become a habit! Whenever a new challenge arises, my sister will now say, "Ok, what's the bright side?" And we'll work it out in our minds until we come up with something and then amazingly, the problem doesn't seem quite so big! I've included a few pages for you to journal about some of your challenges in life, and then stop a moment and think of the bright side and write it down. That is exactly how this little book began.

My challenge _____
_____
_____

The bright side _____
_____
_____
_____

My challenge _____
_____
_____

The bright side _____
_____
_____
_____

Finding the Bright Side

My challenge _____

_____

_____

The bright side _____

_____

_____

_____

My challenge _____

_____

_____

The bright side _____

_____

_____

_____

Finding the Bright Side

My challenge _____
_____
_____
_____

The bright side _____
_____
_____
_____

My challenge _____
_____
_____
_____

The bright side _____
_____
_____
_____
_____

Finding the Bright Side

My challenge _____

_____

_____

The bright side _____

_____

_____

_____

My challenge _____

_____

_____

The bright side _____

_____

_____

_____

_____

My challenge _____
_____
_____
_____

The bright side _____
_____
_____
_____
_____

My challenge _____
_____
_____
_____

The bright side _____
_____
_____
_____
_____

Finding the Bright Side

My challenge _____
_____
_____

The bright side _____
_____
_____
_____

My challenge _____
_____
_____

The bright side _____
_____
_____
_____

My challenge _____

_____

_____

_____

The bright side _____

_____

_____

_____

My challenge _____

_____

_____

_____

The bright side _____

_____

_____

_____

_____

Finding the Bright Side

My challenge _____

_____

_____

The bright side _____

_____

_____

_____

My challenge _____

_____

_____

The bright side _____

_____

_____

_____

_____

Finding the Bright Side

My challenge _____
_____
_____
_____

The bright side _____
_____
_____
_____
_____

My challenge _____
_____
_____
_____

The bright side _____
_____
_____
_____
_____

Finding the Bright Side

My challenge _____
_____
_____

The bright side _____
_____
_____
_____

My challenge _____
_____
_____

The bright side _____
_____
_____
_____

Finding the Bright Side

My challenge _____

_____

_____

_____

The bright side _____

_____

_____

_____

My challenge _____

_____

_____

_____

The bright side _____

_____

_____

_____

_____

Finding the Bright Side

My challenge _____

_____

_____

The bright side _____

_____

_____

_____

My challenge _____

_____

_____

The bright side _____

_____

_____

_____

_____

Finding the Bright Side

My challenge _____

_____

_____

_____

The bright side _____

_____

_____

_____

_____

My challenge _____

_____

_____

_____

The bright side _____

_____

_____

_____

_____

Finding the Bright Side

My challenge _____

_____

_____

_____

The bright side _____

_____

_____

_____

_____

My challenge _____

_____

_____

_____

The bright side _____

_____

_____

_____

_____

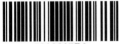

Made in the USA
Charleston, SC
26 May 2010